A NOTE ON LANGUAGE:

throughout this zine you will read phrases like "people with cycles" or "people with eggs" or "people with sperm." this may be a new way of talking for you, and that's okay! you might also be wondering, "why don't they just say girls & women or boys & men?" we use these special phrases because we want to respect that not all girls & women have a uterus and not all people who have a uterus are girls and women. there are lots of different bodies, genders, and identities, and we want this info to be inclusive, safe, and educational for everyone!

why talk about periods & cycles at all?!

have your parents & teachers started talking to you about how your body is changing or about getting your first period? are you curious about why this is an important topic? even though you may have been told that all of this is about "becoming a woman"* it's actually about so much more (and it's much more interesting than that!). getting your first (or second, or third) period — in other words, starting to have a menstrual cycle — is one part of a new journey to becoming a young adult (and yes, maybe someday, to have babies). we want you to learn about these cycles so that you know how awesome & amazing your body is. plus, having cycles means lots of changes are happening, and just like you wouldn't want to get in a car and start driving without knowing how, it's super helpful to understand your cycles.

* if you have a body with a uterus and are feeling like these cycles go against your sense of self or identity, that's okay too. it might be good to talk to a doctor or therapist or other adult you trust about how to feel good in your body as it starts to change.

DID YOU KNOW?

the uterus is the strongest muscle by weight and it exerts the strongest force of any muscle!

internal parts

before we dive deeper into periods & menstrual cycles, let's take a look at the uterus (which is part of our anatomy we can't see) and all of its different parts.

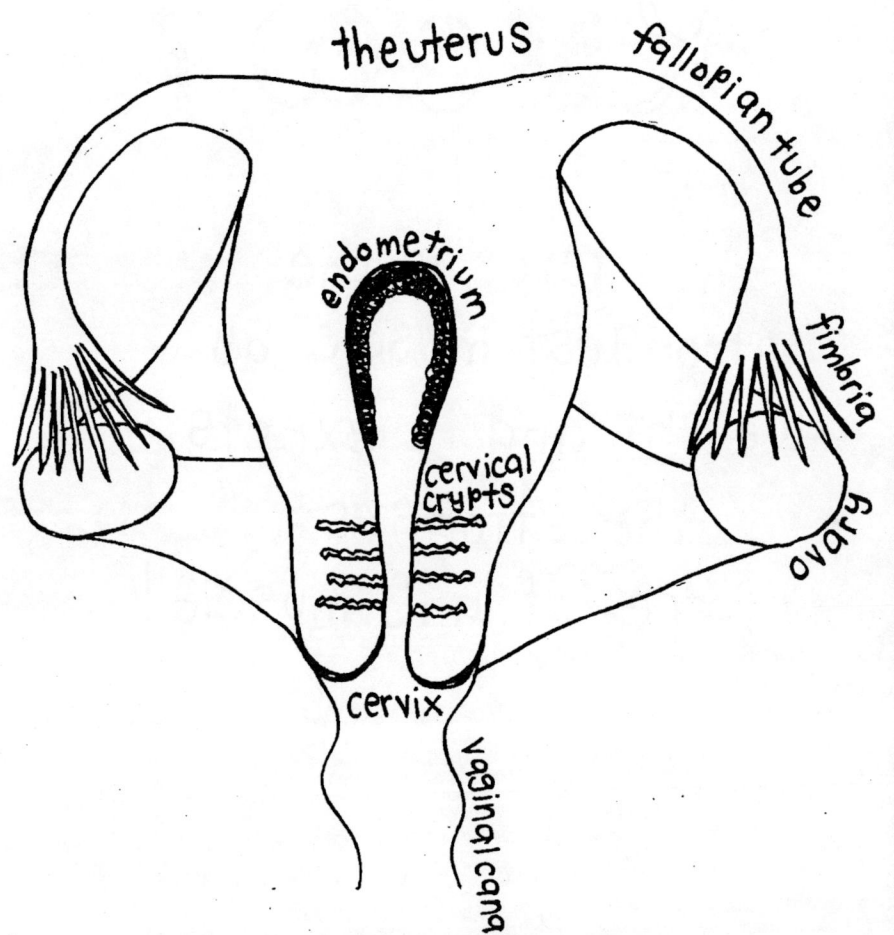

the uterus: the uterus is where your period blood comes from and also where babies can grow. it's about the size and shape of a pear or lemon.

endometrium: just like the inside of your coat has a lining, your uterus has a cozy & plush lining too, called the endometrium. it's made of blood & tissue that build up every cycle. if an egg is fertilized, it will travel to the endometrium and burrow in. if the egg is not fertilized, the endometrium is shed (meaning it leaves your uterus by exiting the cervix and then vagina).

ovary: you have two almond sized ovaries which contain all your eggs!

fallopian tube: you also have two tiny tubes that connect to the uterus. sperm use these little tunnels to get to the egg and a fertilized egg uses them to get inside of the uterus.

fimbria: the fimbriae (plural of fimbria) are like little brooms that hover over your ovaries. they swish against the outside of the ovary in order to catch the tiny egg released at ovulation. if the fimbriae weren't there to sweep up the egg, it would go floating out into your body and never be seen again!

cervix: the opening of the uterus into the vaginal canal. this is where period blood comes out of, where babies (usually) come out of, and where cervical fluid comes out of.

cervical crypts: tunnels that line the cervix & where cervical fluid is made!

vaginal canal: the tunnel that leads from the cervix into the outside world!

what is a menstrual cycle?

you've probably heard all about periods but what's this other thing called a menstrual cycle (or cycle, for short)

		☆ 1	2	3	4	5
6	7	8	9	10	11	12
13	14	15	16	17	18	19
20	21	22	23	24 ☆	25	26
27	28	29	30	31		

if you start your period (bleeding) on the 1st, and another period on the 24th, then your cycle was 23 days. the menstrual cycle is the length of time from one period to the next.

there is so much more going on during your cycle other than periods, though. the main event of your cycle is actually something called ovulation, which is when one of your ovaries releases an egg (sometimes two eggs). the whole goal of the cycle is to release this egg. sometimes during ovulation (which happens once per cycle), the egg meets up with sperm. this is called fertilization. if this egg + sperm grows in the uterus for about 9 months it will be a baby! if the egg doesn't meet up with sperm, the egg dies and a couple weeks later is shed when you have your period.

although young people with cycles don't ovulate very often during the first 2-3 years, by age 18 you'll ovulate about 50% of the time, and by age 25, about 85% of the time.* right now, your body is learning how to ovulate. its a big new skill, and it takes a few years to get good at it.

* from www.acog.org "menstruation in girls and adolescents: using the menstrual cycle as a vital sign"

REVIEW ♡

Period: days of bleeding (also known as menstruation).

Cycle: the length of time between periods, often with ovulation occurring sometime in the middle of the cycle.

Ovulation: when an egg is released by your ovary.

the Uterus: a super strong muscle in your body where period blood comes from (and where babies can grow).

the Ovaries: containers for all of your eggs.

DID YOU KNOW?

you were born with about one million eggs in your ovaries!

Sex and Pregnancy

remember how the uterus is where a baby grows, and that it all starts with the egg getting "fertilized" by sperm? well, now we know where the egg comes from (the ovary!), but what about the sperm? how does it get there? the egg and sperm can meet a few different ways. one way is when two people, one who has eggs and the other who has sperm "have sex." sex can mean lots of different things, but in this case it means that two people get their bodies close together in a way that allows sperm from the penis to go inside the vagina, travel through the cervix & uterus, and meet up with the egg from the ovary. another way to fertilize an egg is to help the egg and sperm meet without having sex, like using special tools and maybe the help of a doctor or midwife.

there is so much more to say about sex and bodies, and we'll explain a little more later.

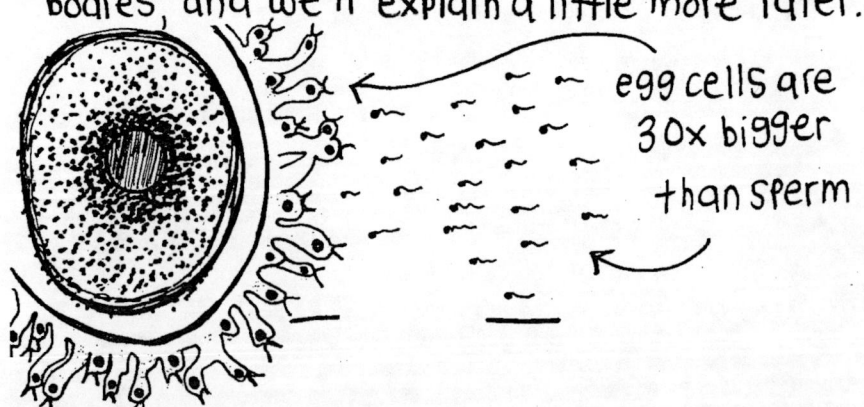

egg cells are 30x bigger than sperm

red flow & clear flow

can you imagine not knowing if you were on your period? impossible — it's so obvious, right? after all, it's RED. one way of talking about it is calling it "the red flow." but did you know there's another kind of flow during your cycle that is just as easy to spot if you know what to look for? it's the "clear flow!" remember the big important event called ovulation, where the ovary releases an egg? your cervix knows when ovulation is about to happen, and as that time gets close, it makes an amazing thing called cervical fluid, or clear flow (it's called that because it often looks clear, wet, and even stretchy. it can also look like lotion, milk, or glue). the clear flow is the only way that sperm can find the egg at ovulation — without it, they die and can't go anywhere. once you start paying attention, the clear flow will be too obvious to miss. even if you haven't started your period yet, you can still notice the clear flow as your ovaries gear up for trying to ovulate.

EXTERNAL PARTS and gender identity

unlike the uterus, which is inside of our body, we also have important parts on the outside parts we can see. we call these parts our "external genitalia." but before we learn about these parts it's good to know that there are lots and lots and lots of different ways our external genitalia can look, and lots of different ways we can feel about our bodies.

some people have a vulva, which often includes parts like labia, a clitoris, a vagina opening (we learned about this one!) and a perineum. some people have testes and a penis. often, when a person is born with a vaginal opening we say, "it's a girl!" and when a person is born with a penis we say, "it's a boy!" sometimes people realize later that the gender (boy or girl) they were assigned at birth isn't actually the gender they are or feel like.

and sometimes people are born with parts that don't quite fit into either category perfectly, and that's okay too. for example, a person might be born appearing to be female on the outside, but having mostly male-typical anatomy on the inside. or a person might be born with a larger clitoris, or lacking a vaginal opening, or a small penis, or a scrotum that's divided more like labia.*

usually these people are put in one category or the other, and sometimes have surgeries as a baby, or as they get older. more and more we are using other categories for people's bodies (instead of just girl & boy) like intersex (these bodies aren't exactly what we expect to see, but it doesn't mean anything is wrong), trans or transgender (when someone is called one gender at birth but switches to another later), non-binary (when a person doesn't feel like they fit in either category), or genderfluid (folks who feel that they fit into one category or another at different times).

*from www.insa.org

typical vulva

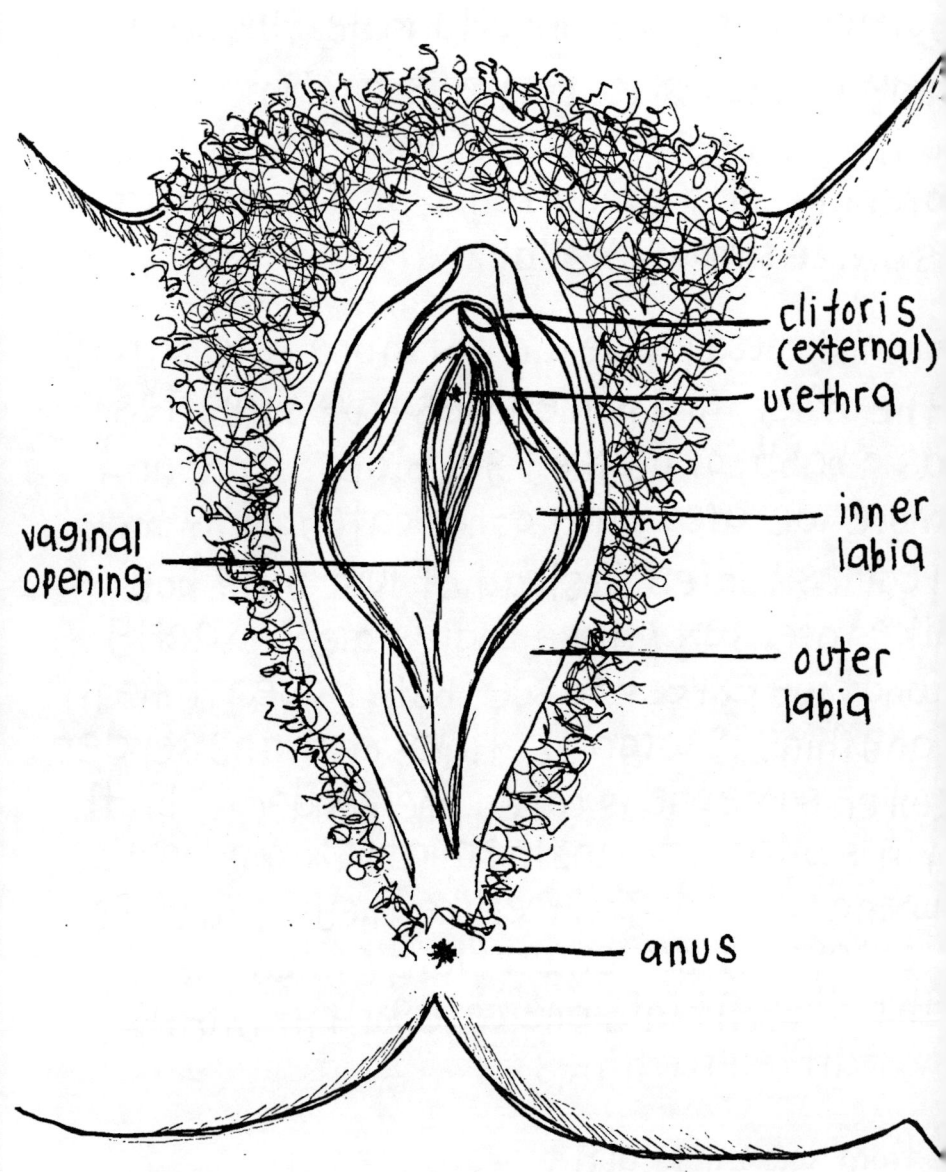

typical penis & testes

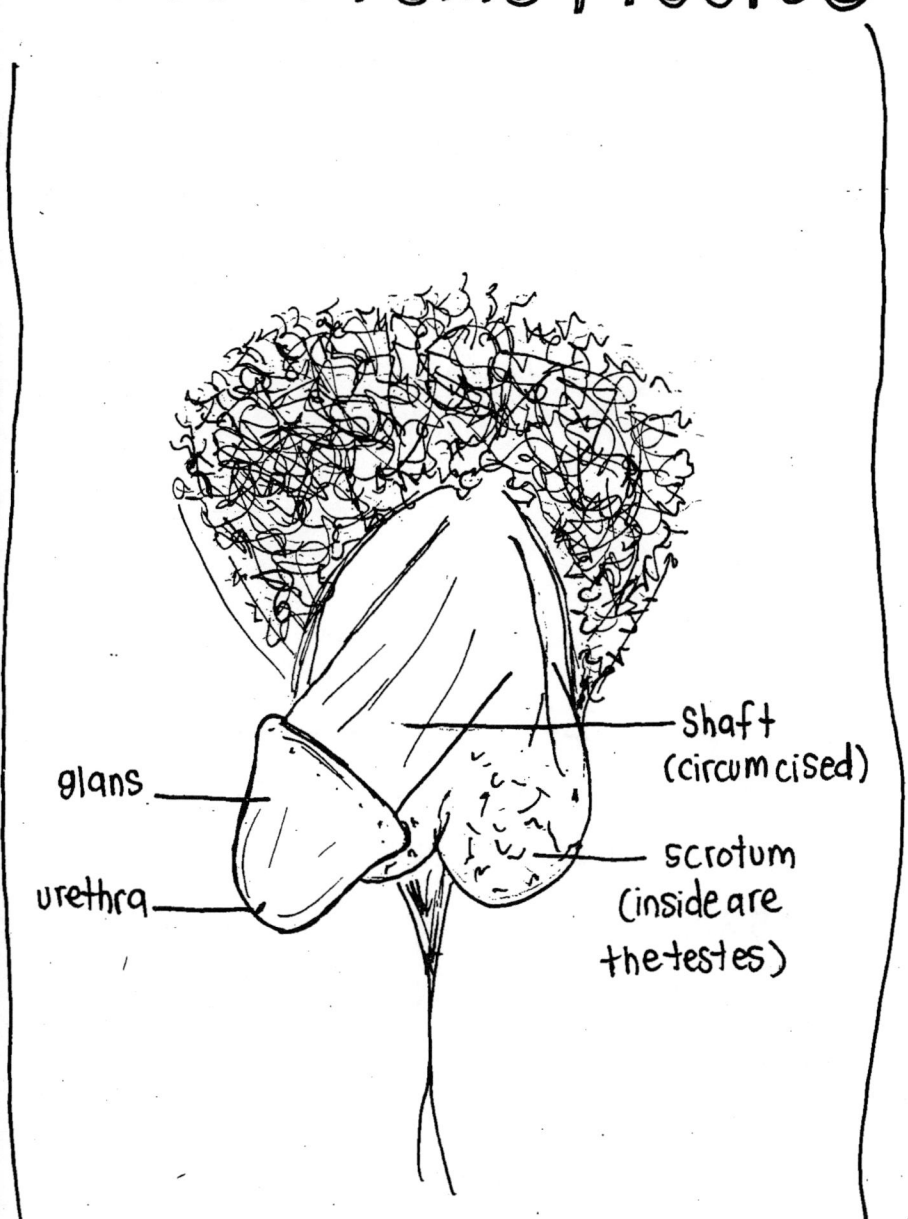

how our bodies grow before we are born!

all fertilized eggs start off the same, no matter if they are going to have a penis or a vulva. around 7 weeks gestation the external genitalia looks like this:

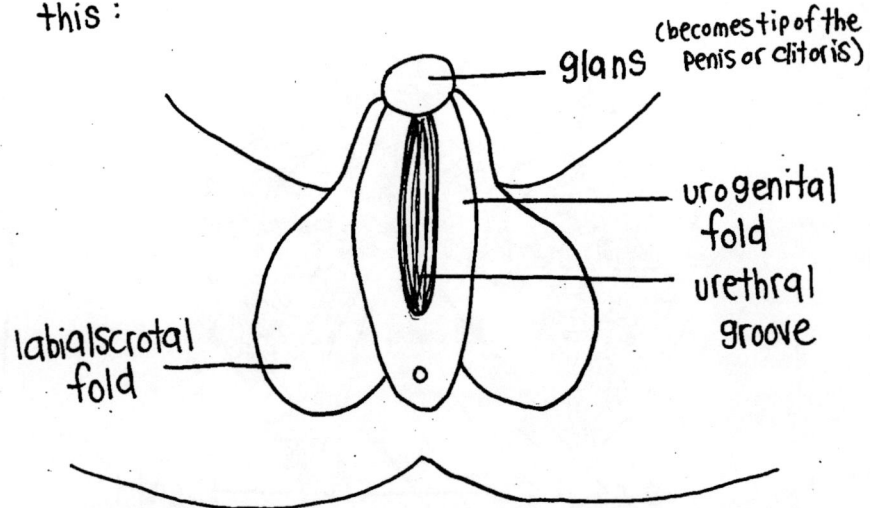

then, around 13 weeks some "differentiation" starts to happen. this just means that some bodies start to look one way (like a vulva), some bodies start to look another way (like a penis), and some bodies aren't quite either (intersex). ultimately, we all have lots of the same parts it's just that they end up looking different. and that's okay! uniqueness is super cool!!

the clitoris

there is one more super special external & internal part that we want to explain a bit more.

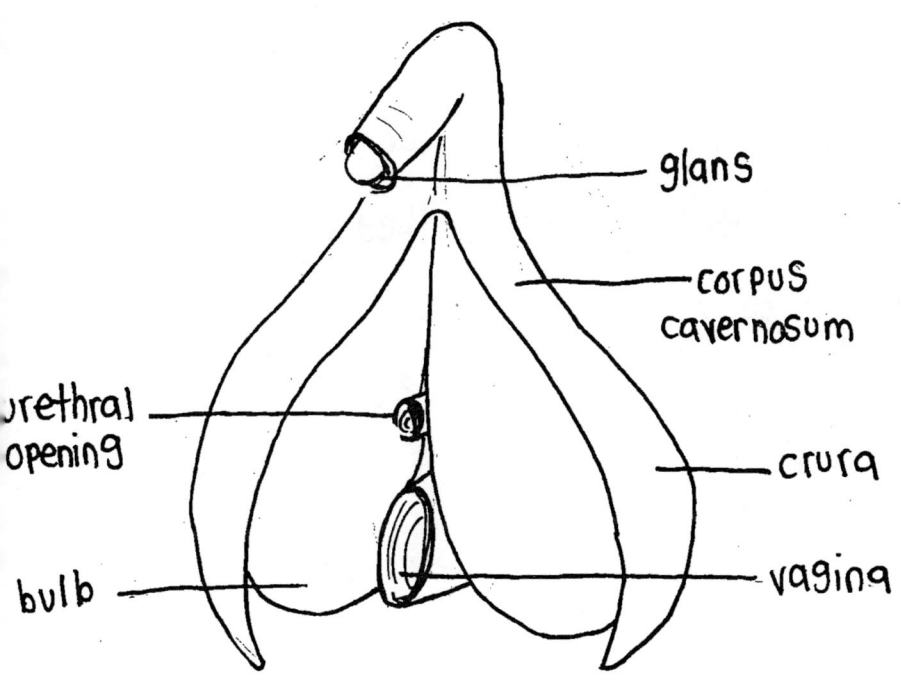

the clitoris is ultra special! know why? it's the only part of your body made just for pleasure! that means it's there to be touched & bring you good feelings. the clitoris actually has 8,000 nerve endings and has parts on both the inside and outside.

REVIEW ♡

clear flow: a special fluid that's made inside the cervix before ovulation (appearing clear, wet, stretchy, like lotion)

sex: when people touch each other's body for pleasure, whether they want to make a baby, to connect emotionally, or just feel good.

fertilization: when an egg joins a sperm.

vulva: all the body parts surrounding (and including!) the vagina.

clitoris: an organ made just for pleasure that starts at the top of the vulva and extends down either side.

intersex: a person who is born with reproductive anatomy that doesn't fit typical definitions of female and male.

DiD YoU KNOW?

the uterus produces special chemicals (hormones) that protect you from heart disease and make you feel happy!

let's talk a little more about sex & sexuality.

we know that sex can mean a lot of different things, but generally, it has to do with people doing things that feel good with their bodies. sexuality is another word word we use when we talk about what we do with our bodies, things we think about, things we want to do with our bodies or with someone else's for pleasure, and how we express ourselves.

one way that some people like to express their sexuality is through masturbation (another new word!) also called self pleasure. this word can also mean a lot of different things, but usually it means someone doing something to their own body in order to feel good. you may already be experimenting with this, or it may be completely new to you.

touching your clitoris, vulva, vagina, or any other part of your body is a-okay. in your bedroom, in the shower, in a private, safe space is the best place to experiment with your body and see what feels good. it's also a good idea to wash your hands before and after touching yourself to prevent irritating sensitive parts of your body.

CONSENT

there are lots of other important things to talk about when it comes to bodies and sex, but here's the bottom line: you get to decide what happens to your body.

what does that mean? one thing that is good to know right away is that you always get to make decisions about who gets to touch your body. if you are ever feeling uncomfortable about the way someone is touching or interacting with your body, you can always say no, or stop. it's really important to tell an adult you trust if this happens.

this might feel really complicated and confusing, so let's break it down into two categories: safe vs. unsafe touch.

SAFE TOUCH means touching that makes you feel cared for, important, or happy, like a pat on the back, a hug from someone you're happy to see, or when someone helps you with an injury, like pulling out a splinter. safe touch is touch that you want, like, and agree to, or need to have in order to help you.

UNSAFE TOUCH means touching that makes you feel scared, bad, or disrespected, such as hitting, holding too tight, not letting go, or touching you in places (like your vulva, breasts, or butt) you don't want someone else to touch. unsafe touch is touch that you don't want, don't like, and don't agree to, or whenever someone tells you to keep it a secret. unsafe touch is never your fault, and you can tell a trusted adult if it happens to you.

REVIEW ♡

masturbation: (or self-pleasure) touching your own clitoris, vulva, or other parts to feel good.

consent: giving and asking for permission to do things with and to each other.

sexuality: how we feel and think about our bodies and other people's bodies, pleasure, and relationships.

these are all really big, important topics, and it's okay to have lots of questions or to be unsure how you feel about it all right now.

let's jump back into the menstrual cycle and learn a little bit more about how it all works.

HORMONES

before we talk about the hormones of the menstrual cycle, let's explain what a hormone even is. a hormone is a kind of messenger that travels all around the body, telling our organs what to do. hormones help us sleep, digest food, feel emotions, grow skin, and a million other things. hormones are also the very thing that makes us have cycles!

the hormones that create the menstrual cycle are made in two places, the brain & the ovaries. at the start of a new cycle, the brain "wakes up" the ovaries by creating a hormone called follicle stimulating hormone, or FSH. the brain talks back & forth with the ovaries and they start to create estrogen, which helps grow a handful of eggs inside the ovaries. estrogen makes us feel excited and energetic!

eventually one egg grows big & beautiful and becomes the chosen one, while all the others die off. then, when the brain sends down a big supply of another hormone, called luteinizing hormone or LH, the egg bursts out of the ovary and travels into the fallopian tube, where it will live just 12-24 hours. this is called ovulation! right after that, a new hormone called progesterone is made (in the ovary), which makes us feel calm, cozy, & warm (it raises our temperature) if the egg is not fertilized, all our hormones drop after about two weeks, we start to menstruate, and a whole new cycle starts again!

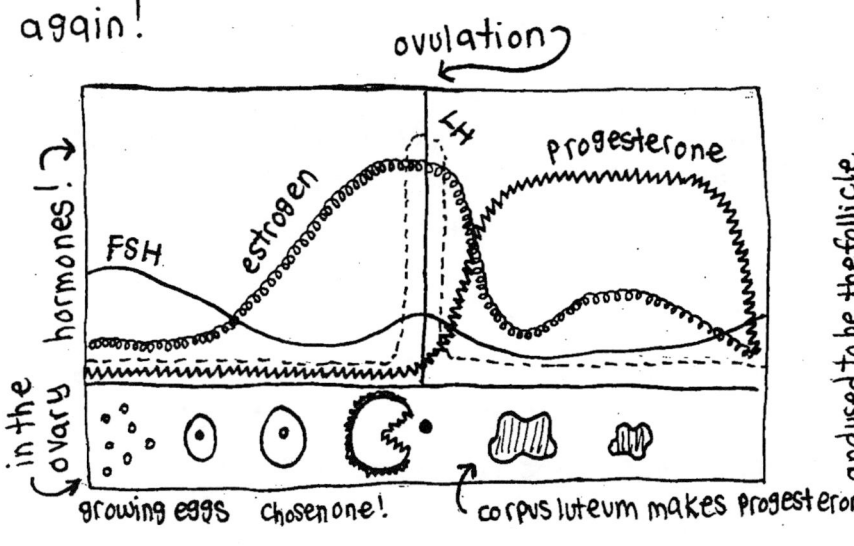

seasons of the cycle
☀ 💧 🍃 ❄

the menstrual cycle is one kind of cycle. there are lots of other cycles too! can you think of any? the solar or lunar cycles, the seasons of the year? what if we pretend like each phase of the cycle were a season:

WINTER we like to wear warm clothes and not be busy when it's wet & cold. during menstruation, we often like to be warm, quiet, & restful. animals hibernate and stay warm & dry.

SPRING the earth wakes up! birds & plants are excited and we are happy to have warmth return. before ovulation we often feel excited & energetic and we do things like play outside, be creative and make music & art, or have sleepovers.

SUMMER we love to relax, chill out, & enjoy life! nature is full of green leaves & flowers. during & after ovulation, we often feel calm, positive, happy.

FALL trees start to shed their leaves, animals prepare nests with food & warmth for the coming winter. just before menstruation, we often want to rest more, eat certain foods, and prepare to get cozy for the "wintertime" of the cycle.

DID YOU KNOW?

Periods are the only type of bleeding in humans that does not mean injury! in fact, periods show us that our bodies are working just right! periods are like a super power!

what's "normal" when you first start having cycles?

you might have heard that your cycle will usually be 28 days long, or that your period will last about 5 days. those numbers refer to averages for adults who cycle, not young people. remember that having cycles is a huge new project for your body, and it takes a few (or many!) years to start having predictable cycles. here are some guidelines for what's more or less average for anyone under 18:

- your cycles are between 21 – 45 days long
- you get your period at least once every 3 months
- period pain is mild & doesn't affect your activities
- you don't feel dizzy, nauseous, weak, or light-headed while on your period.
- your bleeding lasts 4 – 8 days
- you don't have to change your pad or tampon more than every 1 – 2 hours
- if you experience period pain or heavy bleeding that makes you double over, throw up, or feel weak, get a trusted adult to help you — that is not just "how periods are" and is cause for concern

how can you tell when you're going to get your period for the first time?

* * * * * * * * * * * * * * *

there are a few signs you can look for. usually you'll get your first period about 2-3 years after you start developing breasts. you'll also probably notice some cervical fluid on your underwear, which can look like a wet spot, like dried paste, or like a white patch. that means your body is starting to think about ovulating soon, and your cervix is starting to make the clear flow! if you see some really wet, stretchy stuff, that means you're getting even closer to periods! you might see some spotting (a very light amount of blood that you see just once, or not very often) or feel some light cramping in your uterus (think stomach area, but much lower).

NORMAL & ABNORMAL SECRETIONS

you know the difference between clear mucus from your nose after a single sneeze, and green gunk from a bad cold, right? your vagina gives signals about your health in the same way. it might sound weird, but just like you can tell when your nose, eyes, ears, and mouth are healthy by the kinds of secretions they make, you can tell if what you see at your vulva is normal too. you probably already know how your vulva feels and smells everyday. maybe you've even noticed some vaginal secretions (like white stuff on your underwear, or stretchy fluid when you wipe with toilet paper). all of this is normal! if there's a problem though, your body will make other fluids that let you know something's not right. how do you tell the difference between them?

NORMAL:

- slight moisture or a bit of white sticky stuff. the vagina is never completely dry and there will usually be something there all the time.
- cervical fluid (clear flow): white, sticky, pasty, watery, clear, stretchy, creamy, looks like raw egg white
- period blood: dark red, light red, pinkish, brownish
- some small clots
- spotting (a light amount of blood) that happens just before your period starts, after it ends, or right around ovulation.

ABNORMAL:

- discharge that looks clumpy or like cottage cheese
- discharge that is green or grey tinged or foamy
- discharge along with redness, pain, swelling, or itching around your vulva
- big clots in your period blood (a clot is like a round blob) that are bigger than a quarter, along with feeling faint, dizzy, nauseous, or weak
- bleeding that is black, grey, or smells bad

→ CYCLE ISSUES

(this is a short list for quick reading! if you see something from the abnormal category on the previous page, chat with an adult or doctor you trust! if you want to learn more about these cycle issues check out our resource list for a link to a happy-cycles guide!)

PERIOD PAIN: a little pain that comes & goes and doesn't cause you to stop your normal activities is okay. but if you can't get up, can't move, feel like you're going to throw up or pass out from pain, that's not okay. a myth about periods is that it's normal for them to make you feel terrible — that's just not true! preventing period pain is kind of a big topic, and we recommend you talk to a trusted adult for help. you could ask them to research some things to help avoid pain, like magnesium, omega-3, cramp bark, or to make sure really healthy foods are available to eat (because junk food = more cramps!).

HEAVY BLEEDING:
if you're soaking through a pad or tampon every 2 hours, and if you also feel weak or dizzy, you might be bleeding too much. ask an adult about ibuprofen (this works quick to slow bleeding, chlorophyll, or capsicum to stop heavy bleeding. and maybe check in with a doctor to see if there is an underlying problem.

REALLY BAD / SAD MOODS:
it's okay and normal to feel all your emotions, no matter how strong! letting yourself feel a bad mood will help it pass. what do you need when you feel angry/upset? do you need a long bath? do you need to be alone? do you need to sit in the sun, write, or play the drums? try making a list! you can also boost emotional health with food, sleep, friends, therapy, and other things.

SORE BREASTS:
you can try massaging your breasts with violet oil or balm, using a heating pad or hot water bottle, or certain supplements like evening primrose. tight bras can make sore breasts worse, so consider not wearing one at all or one that doesn't squeeze too tight.

menstrual PRODUCTS
(cup!) (pad!)

now that you know about your red flow, you may also be wondering about the different options for collecting this flow.

some options are disposable (like pads & tampons), which means you use them once and then throw them away. these can be really nice if you are out & about for the day and need to change your pad or tampon a couple times. if possible, it's best to use organic pads & tampons. some of the other brands use harsh chemicals like bleach or fragrances that can be uncomfortable or cause problems. we listed some places to order organic menstrual products in the resources, or if you live near a food co-op or health food store, you should be able to find them locally.

some other options for catching your red flow are reusable pads and something called a menstrual cup, both of which can be used cycle after cycle.

reusable pads are made of cloth, and some people like the way they feel better than disposables. they also create a lot less waste, which is good for the earth! you can bring a few with you when you leave the house and bring a little plastic bag for when you want to change them. at the end of the day just rinse them in the sink and wash them with the rest of your laundry!

menstrual cups are a little different — some people have a harder time getting them inside the vagina at first and that's okay. once you get the hang of them you can keep them in for 10-12 hours. they are shaped like a little cup, are usually made of soft, flexible silicone, and sit right up at the cervix to catch the blood. when you take them out, you can just dump the blood in the toilet, rinse the cup in the sink or just wipe it with toilet paper, and use it again. it's good to wash the cup regularly with soap or pour boiling water on it to help keep it clean.

keeping track

one way to learn more about your unique cycle is to track it! it's like doing scientific research on YOU! tracking your periods will give you an idea of when to expect the next one. you'll start to notice clues that tell you what's going on with your cycle, like that you always feel moody or crave certain foods at the same time every cycle. there are a few different things you can track, and you can pay attention to all of them or pick & choose which ones feel useful.

Period! (red flow): even if you think all of this is super boring, it's a good idea to keep track of when you have a period, how long it lasted, and the flow (heavy, medium, or light).

Cervical fluid! (clear flow): make notes about clear, slippery, fluid, what it feels like, how much, etc

other symptoms!: breast tenderness, moods, cravings, emotions, dreams, acne, energy

here are some different ways you can track your cycle:

★ you can make a note in your phone (if you have a phone!) about when your period starts and how long it lasts.

★ you can use a paper chart to write down all the things you notice throughout your cycle, like periods, cervical fluid, spotting, mood changes, and more (it's like a journal, art, and science project in one!).

★ you can try out some different period charting apps. helloclue.com is a good one we recommend!

★ buy or make a calendar for each month. make up your own special code, or use this one =

* bleeding (*** heavy, ** medium * light)

(*) spotting

☽ cervical fluid

↑ high energy!

↓ low energy

resource list

- scarleteen.com
- cycle savvy by toni weschler
- sex is a funny word by cory silverberg
- it's perfectly normal by robie h. harris
- putacupinit.com/quiz (menstrual cup guide)
- cora.life or mylola.com (organic products)
- glad rags or luna pads (cloth pads)
- isna.org (intersex info)
- our bodies ourselves
- cycle-wise.com/freebies (healthy cycles guide & PDF cycle chart!)

discussion questions

whether you're reading through this alone, with a friend, family member, mentor or trusted adult, these questions are for you!

- what's the scariest thing about getting your first period?

- what's exciting about getting your first period?

- do you want to do something special when you get your period for the first time? a special dinner? a gift? a big hug?

- what words instantly come to mind when you think about periods?

- what else do you want to know about periods, cycles, or bodies after reading this zine?

SUBSCRIBE TO EVERYTHING WE PUBLISH!

Do you love what Microcosm publishes?

Do you want us to publish more great stuff?

Would you like to receive each new title as it's published?

Subscribe as a BFF to our new titles and we'll mail them all to you as they are released!

$13-30/mo, pay what you can afford!

microcosmpublishing.com/bff

...AND HELP US GROW YOUR SMALL WORLD!

More reproductive health from Ashley Hartman Annis

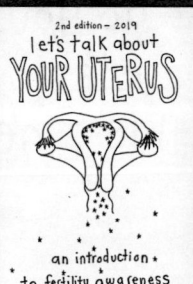